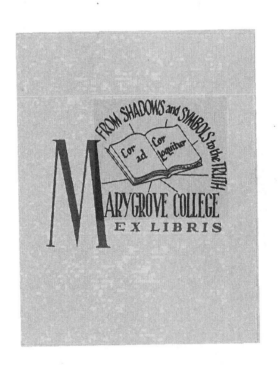

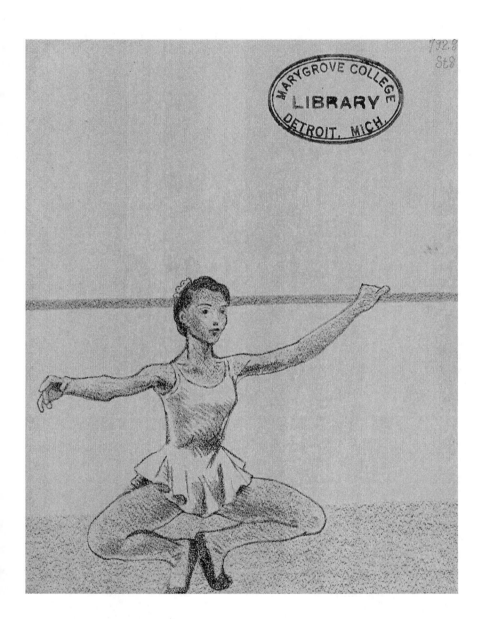

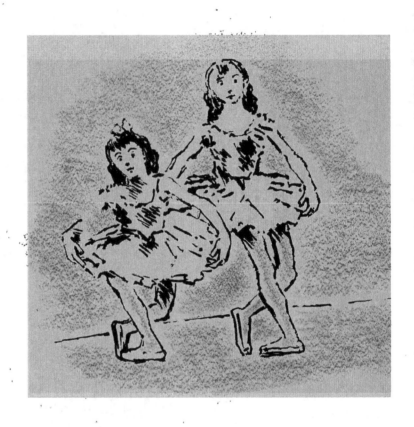

FIRST PRINTING
Printed in the United States of America
by the Polygraphic Company of America, Inc.
Published in Canada by Ambassador Books, Ltd.,
Toronto 1, Ontario
Library of Congress Catalog Card Number: 53-10259

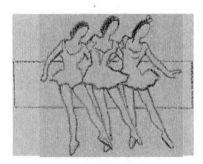

My grateful thanks are given to Arnold Haskell, Director of the Sadler's Wells Ballet School, not only for every word he has written about ballet training, but for his accessibility. In the many years I have known him I have never asked him a question on ballet matters which he has not found time to answer, fully and of course illuminatingly.

*Noel Streatfeild*

I should like to thank dancers Electa Arenal, who patiently posed for the drawings, and Phyllis Swirin, who did most of the research. I also appreciate the help of the Dance Notation Bureau, who were kind enough to supply the floor plans of part of the Third Movement of *Symphonie Concertante*, by Georges Balanchine, which appear on page 87.

*Moses Soyer*

# Contents

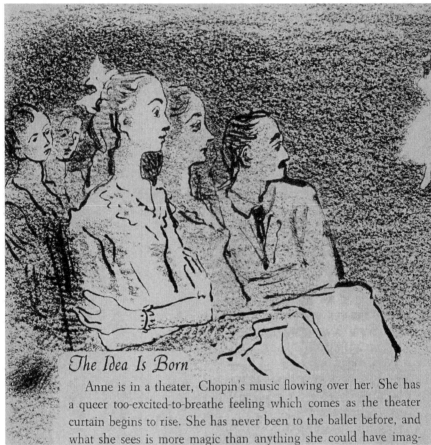

## The Idea Is Born

Anne is in a theater, Chopin's music flowing over her. She has a queer too-excited-to-breathe feeling which comes as the theater curtain begins to rise. She has never been to the ballet before, and what she sees is more magic than anything she could have imagined. There is a grove of trees with a ruined building half hidden in them. The moon is shining; the world is misty and green. At

8

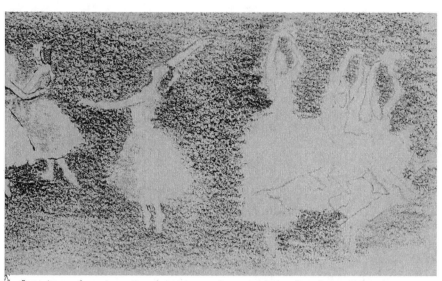

first Anne doesn't notice the trees or the moonlight, for she is staring at the first ballet dancers she has ever seen.

The stage is full of girls all dressed alike in filmy white dresses that stop just above their ankles. There are white flowers around their heads, and little silver wings at their waists. Among the trees is a group of four dancers, three girls and one man. One of the girls wears a little pink rose on the front of her dress.

Anne finds the dancers puzzling, for their faces don't look real. They seem to be dancing in their sleep. Even their arms don't look real. They move as if there were no bones in them. The music changes, and a girl dances alone. It changes again. Now it is the girl with the pink rose who is dancing.

9

At first Anne shows no sign that anything has happened to her, for she is past speech. How could she know that legs can do the things she sees legs doing? How could she know that arms can ripple like waves ruffled by a breeze?

Father, looking at Anne's rapt face, nudges Mother and whispers that he is glad they took her to the ballet, though it is not what he would have chosen for himself. He guessed Anne would enjoy it, bless her! Neither Father nor Mother has any idea that they have lit a flame in Anne's heart which nothing can put out— that the Anne who went into the theater has come out quite a different person.

When Anne got home, home was not the place it had been, either. Was it possible all she had wanted that morning was the usual kind of fun? Anne said nothing about her feelings, for she was afraid of being laughed at. You are silent when you are nursing a dream, and mothers are apt to mistake silence for sickness, so Anne was put to bed for a while. She had to suffer for her secret. But the secret wouldn't stay inside her; it began growing and coming to the surface. When she was sure no one was around, she tried to dance as the girl with the rose danced. She struggled painfully onto the tips of her square-toed school shoes. She waved her arms before her mirror. She struggled—and a very noisy struggle it was—to float from one side of her bedroom to the other. It was these efforts that forced her secret into the open.

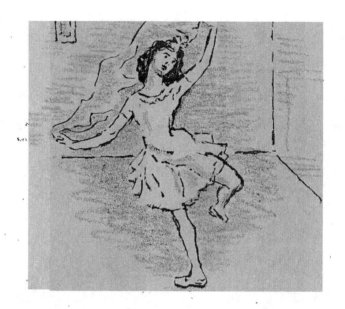

## Too Old or Too Tall

Anne had spoken. She had told her mother, "I am going to be a dancer." Mother had repeated with disbelief, "She wants to be a dancer." But the words were said! They were hanging in the living room almost as visible as washing on a line. Mother could see that Anne really wanted this more than anything else in the world. The possibilities now had to be talked out.

The first thing Anne's family had to consider was how old Anne should be to start training to be a dancer. There is no definite answer to this. Girls have succeeded who did not take a

11

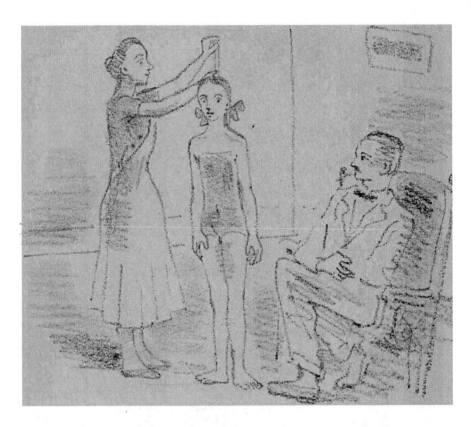

lesson until they were in their teens, but they are the exceptions, and only they could say how much they suffered by starting late. Most ballet schools specify ten as the right age to start serious training, though a few take pupils who have passed their ninth birthday. Of course this does not mean that Anne could not have gone to an ordinary dancing school ever since she was a little girl, but for formal training, the family learned, ten is about the best age to begin.

The next thing they had to think about was Anne's height. Tall girls have become fine ballet dancers, but very few of them have done so, for being tall is a great disadvantage. When Anne first heard this she said, "I don't believe height matters a bit, look at...," and then she named a tall ballerina. What Anne had forgotten is that a dancer seen·on the stage looks far taller than she really is. She has to dance with men who never stand on their *pointes* (pwahnt), or tips of their toes, while she will often be dancing on hers. If Anne measured the length of her feet, and added it to her height, she could see how tall she would be when she was standing on her toes. Anyway, no matter how Anne might argue, dancing is a doubtful career to choose for a girl who is likely to be tall. Anne's parents could make a pretty good guess as to how tall she would be. If Father's relatives were mostly six-footers, and all Mother's family five-foot seven and over, the chances are Anne would not grow up to be a fairy-like little creature of five-foot two. But Anne skipped over these two first hurdles. She was not yet ten, and nobody was tall on either side of her family, so the only problem was: How could her family choose the right ballet school?

## Beware the Witch

Though neither Anne nor her family had any idea of it, the choice of her ballet teacher was so important it is impossible to exaggerate what it meant to her future. In fairy stories there are witches who wait to clutch children and either eat them or turn them into toads. In real life greedy, unprincipled ballet teachers are real witches. Instead of eating children, witch ballet teachers lure dollars out of their fathers' pockets for lessons. They train the girls so badly that within a very short time the bones of their feet are thrown out of place, and any chance they had of becoming dancers is finished for good. In order to produce fast "results," unprepared children are taught to get up and dance on the tips of their toes.

No girl can profit from ballet exercises until she has learned to stand properly. Dancing on the toes should only begin after months of hard work, when the feet are ready for blocked ballet shoes. The pupils of poor dancing teachers wear blocked shoes far too soon, and perform difficult steps on the soft bones of their untrained feet. They usually end up with badly misshapen feet. It is hard for a girl to be cooed over and perhaps called "a baby Pavlova," and then find herself at the age of eleven with nothing to show for all the time and money spent but crippled feet! This is the danger Anne's parents had to guard against.

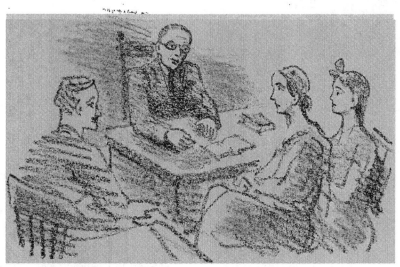

## A Good Dancing Teacher

Anne's father and mother had common sense. They did not know any dancers, but they remembered that the principal of Anne's school was a wise man with many acquaintances. They went to him with their problem. If Anne was determined to dance, was there any teacher nearby whom his friends who knew about dancing could recommend?

The answer took time, but in the end a letter arrived from a man the principal knew. Anne was lucky. She lived in a small community, and there was no good teacher nearby, but in a big town not far away there was a fine teacher called Madame Natalie.

She had joined the Monte Carlo Russian Ballet when she was fifteen, and later danced with the Sadlers' Wells Company in London. She came to America with the troupe, and when they returned to England she stayed in America to be married. Madame. Natalie now had her own ballet school.

At the bottom of the letter there was a footnote. "Your little Anne and her family must not be disappointed if Madame Natalie will not take her. She trains only a few pupils, and each must show real promise."

That footnote made Father and Mother angry. "Must not be disappointed, indeed!" Who did this Madame Natalie think she was, anyway? They would have their child study with her if it were the last thing they did. But Father and Mother soon calmed down. Back Mother went to Anne's principal to thank him for finding out about Madame Natalie, and to ask if he would write and arrange for her to see Anne. Also, what were the right clothes for Anne to wear at the interview?

Father, determined not to spoil Anne's chances, told Mother to get whatever was needed, and not to let a dollar or two stand in the way. But Madame Natalie's reply said that no special clothes were needed. She would see Anne in her studio the following Wednesday. Anne should wear an ordinary school dress. If she had some soft practice shoes she should bring them, but on no account should her parents buy new ones.

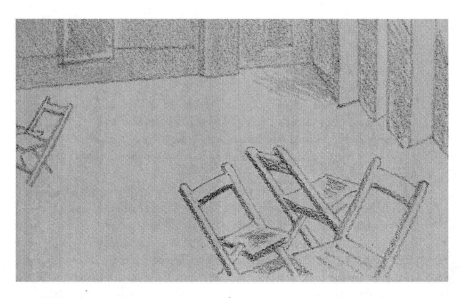

## The Interview

Goodness knows what Anne and her Mother expected Madame Natalie's studio to look like, but certainly not a bit the sort of room it was. They saw a great barnlike place painted off-white, with a few tired-looking chairs propped against the walls, a seedy upright piano at one end, two huge wall mirrors and, around three sides of the room, a railing called the *barre*.

Madame Natalie had black hair parted in the middle and gathered into a bun at her neck. She wore a plain full-skirted black dress, pink tights, pink ballet shoes, and she carried a long stick. Her most noticeable features were her huge dark eyes, which

17

ran over Anne as if she had seen through Anne's skin in one glance, and was examining her bones.

After she said "How do you do," Madame Natalie told Mother to sit down, and asked Anne to take off her shoes and socks. Then, slowly and carefully, she examined Anne's feet. She made no comment about them, so Anne and her mother could only hope they would do.

Madame then told Anne to put on her socks and come with her into the middle of the room. Anne had been captivated by Madame from the first moment she saw her, and would have suffered agonies to please her. Actually what she wanted was not difficult at all. Madame turned out her feet almost parallel, with the front heel to the toe of the back foot and the back heel close to the toe of the front foot. She told Anne to do the same, and then jump in the air, changing feet while off the ground. Then Madame led her to the *barre* and told her to copy what she did. Anne had to bend

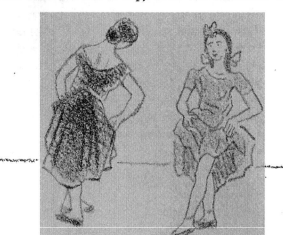

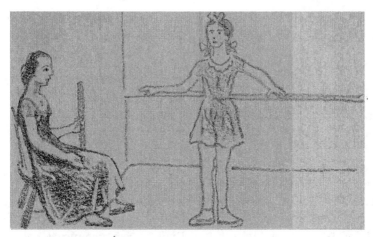

way down with her toes very turned out. Holding onto the *barre* with one hand, she had to lift first one leg and then the other as high as she could without straining. Then she was told to sit down.

Madame sat down with Anne and her mother and began to talk. Anne, she said, was completely untrained, and it was impossible to tell if she would make a dancer or not. All Madame could say was that she had well-shaped feet and a good build for a dancer. It was important to be sure Anne and her parents knew what ballet training really meant.

Madame told Anne to sniff. Could she smell anything? Anne could smell sweat, and said so. People were inclined to think that dancing was a lovely art, Madame went on, and that it must be nice for a girl to learn, but actually dancing was terribly hard work. She herself must have sweated quarts of water since her first lesson, and that was true of every good dancer.

19

"One of my duties as a dancing teacher," Madame said, "is to try to persuade girls like Anne *not* to learn to dance. If she studies with me, there will be little time for the fun most girls have. It will mean work, work, work. What's more, in another profession I might be able to tell you all this sacrifice is worth while, for in the end Anne will be able to repay you by making a lot of money. In the dancing world, however, it is very doubtful."

Madame looked hard at Mother as she went on: "I think no life holds more heartbreak than a dancer's. Her professional life is short, and she cannot be sure of getting a job once she is trained. America has shown that ballet dancers can and should be used in musical shows, and there are other kinds of dancing that Anne might consider if she is not the right type for a ballet company, but there are not many openings. Of course if she is very talented— and lucky—she can become a member of the *corps de ballet*, then a soloist, and someday a ballerina. But I can promise nothing."

Then she turned to Anne. "What do you say? In spite of all I've told you, do you want to come to me and see how you like it? You have two little sisters, I am told. How are you going to feel when you see them eating huge dishes of ice cream and pieces of cake, and you have to say no, because a dancer must not be fat? How are you going to feel when those two little sisters are running off to parties and you stay home to practice?"

Anne said nothing, and Madame laughed. "I can see by the

20

look in your eyes, Anne, that nothing I can say will put you off. Your first sight of a ballet enchanted you. That is how it started with me, too.".

Then, looking very business-like, Madame spoke to Mother. "Very well, I will try her for a year. If at any time during that year I consider she is wasting her time, the lessons will stop. If at the end of the year I can see promise, I will train her." A faraway look came into Madame's eyes as she finished, "And perhaps, who knows, make a dancer of her!"

Before Anne and her mother left, Madame Natalie led Anne into the middle of the room and showed her how to bow, pointing her left leg forward while she stood firmly on the right leg with the foot turned out, and slowly bent her right knee. "That," said Madame Natalie, "is what we call a *révérence.* You will make one at the end of every lesson."

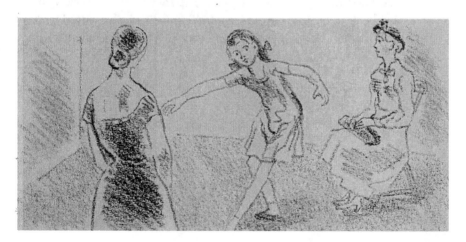

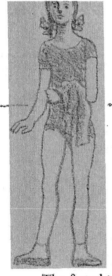

## First Lessons

It was a good thing Anne's love for the ballet was a strong one, or her first dancing classes would surely have worn it down. Her classes took place after school. There were five other girls in Anne's class. The other girls had started some weeks ahead of Anne, but—and this is the discouraging part—they did not seem to have learned much.

The first thing Anne was taught did not seem to her to have anything to do with dancing. She was taught how to breathe.

Madame made "controlled breathing" sound more important than knowing how to use your feet. She showed the girls how to seal the air into their lungs by controlling their diaphragms. Then they had to open their mouths and very slowly let out all the air they had held in. They did this several times during every lesson.

Mother thought the clothes Anne wore for her dancing classes were terrible. There were a pair of soft practice shoes and a garment which looked to her like a bathing suit with sleeves, but which Madame called a leotard (LEE-oh-tahrd). Madame said that for the time being Anne could wear ankle socks. Later on, if

22

she decided Anne was worth training, Anne would need tights and a special tunic. Madame told her always to be sure to bring a clean towel to her classes. Mother sniffed when Madame said that, and told Father later that it was surprising that such a nice-looking woman as Madame could keep on the way she did about sweat.

The word Anne heard most often during her first lessons was "placing." It was only after weeks of struggle that Anne began to understand what it meant.

"Placing" means that every part of the body, from the top of the head to the soles of the feet and the tips of the fingers, is perfectly balanced. Every muscle must be in the right position, no part of the body forced out of line. A dancer must stand easily, with no strain anywhere. It takes a long time to learn how to do this, but when it is learned a real move has been made toward becoming a fine dancer.

The first exercises Anne learned were the five basic positions. She did them holding onto the *barre* to help her balance. Like all other exercises, they are taught using one foot as the "working" foot—the one that moves—and then repeated with the other foot.

Anne heard the word *changé* (shahn-ZHAY) almost as often from her very first lesson. When she was working at the *barre* and the teacher said, "*Changé*, everyone!" it meant turning around, holding the *barre* with the other hand, and doing the same exercise the reverse way to learn to use both feet equally well.

23

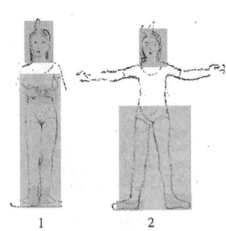

1   2

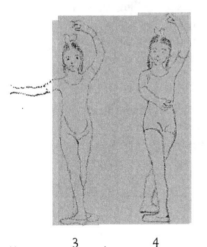

3   4

# BASIC EXERCISES

*First Position*
 Heels together, toes turned out as far as they can go.

*Second Position*
 From first position the right foot slides to the side, leaving room for a practice shoe and a half between the two feet. The weight is balanced evenly on both feet.

*Third Position*
 The right foot is pulled back to the left foot, bringing the right heel against the left instep. Legs and feet are well turned out.

*Fourth Position*
 The right foot slides forward in front of the left foot until the space of a practice shoe and a half separates them. The heel of the front foot must be in line with the toes of the back foot, and both are well turned out.

*Fifth Position*
 The right foot slides straight backward until the toes of the right foot touch the heel of the left and the heel of the right is against the toes of the left. This position is the one most often used in dancing. A great many steps are started from this position.

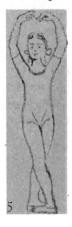

5

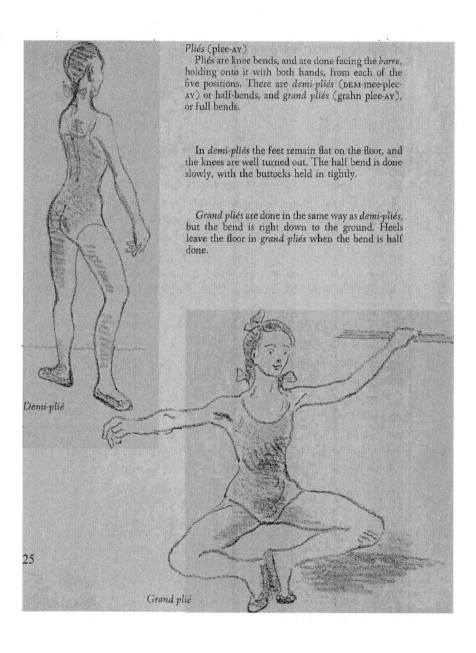

*Pliés* (plee-AY)

Pliés are knee bends, and are done facing the *barre*, holding onto it with both hands, from each of the five positions. There are *demi-pliés* (DEM-mee-plee-AY) or half-bends, and *grand pliés* (grahn plee-AY), or full bends.

In *demi-pliés* the feet remain flat on the floor, and the knees are well turned out. The half bend is done slowly, with the buttocks held in tightly.

*Grand pliés* are done in the same way as *demi-pliés*, but the bend is right down to the ground. Heels leave the floor in *grand pliés* when the bend is half done.

*Demi-plié*

*Grand plié*

## More Lessons

Madame said bends were very important, and all dancers did them every day of their lives. They were very good for limbering the leg muscles and the heels, especially the part of the heel called the Achilles tendon. A well-stretched Achilles tendon was very necessary to a dancer, for it was her springboard. When Madame was present and the girls were practicing bends, her stick was busy pushing out knees and prodding backs. During the first part of the lesson the girls worked at the *barre*, but during the last half they went to the center of the room. There faults of balance showed up very clearly.

Though all lessons were exercises and more exercises, Madame tried to make them interesting. At the end of a class she taught herself, she explained why an exercise had to be learned. She would show a string of little steps from one of the great ballets.

"You see," she would say, "it is no fun just learning exercises and not understanding what they are for. When you see a ballet performed in a theater, I don't want you just to look starry-eyed at the stage thinking how beautiful the dancers are. I want you to see for yourself that the exercises you are learning are the very beginning of dancing, that without them you would be unable to dance at all."

Here are more exercises that Anne learned.

*Battement Tendu . .*
(bat-MAHN tahn-DU)

Feet in fifth position. One foot slides forward and points straight out, not leaving the floor, then returns to fifth position. The exercise is also done to the side and back in the same way.

*Petit Battement* (peh-TEE bat-MAHN)

Starting from fifth position, one foot is lifted, knee well out, to touch the ankle of the supporting foot. Using the knee as a spring, the heel of the working foot beats the ankle of the supporting foot quickly, first in front, then behind.

*Battement Frappé* (bat-MAHN frap-PAY)

From fifth position one foot is raised to the ankle of the supporting foot, keeping the knee well turned out. The working foot is pushed straight forward, brushing the floor, until the leg is straight and the toes are just off the floor. Then it returns quickly to the ankle. This is done to the side and back as well.

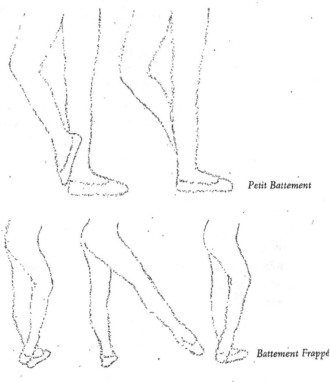

*Petit Battement*

*Battement Frappé*

**Fifth Position**

Anne was also taught to stand on one leg. Before she tried it this seemed so easy that she thought it was ridiculous to have to learn how. The funny thing was, she found, that lifting a leg off the ground while she held the *barre* was hard. This was so partly because the foot that stayed on the ground had to be turned out as nearly as possible at an angle of forty-five degrees. In that first term Anne never managed to stand properly on one leg while holding the *barre*. She could not help bending while she did it, and often her free arm looked stiff as a twig on a tree.

Each evening when she came home Anne tried to tell Father and Mother what she had learned. She showed them the five positions, she tried to make them feel the correct placing, and she offered to teach them bends and her other exercises, but neither of them wanted to learn. Father said you couldn't teach an old dog new tricks, and Mother said Anne had better hold off till the babies were old enough to learn. Anne tried to make Father stand on one leg, but he couldn't.

He said he thought it would be more of a help if he spent his time putting up a *barre*. He fixed a *barre* on the wall, near the entrance hall. Until it was up Anne had done her daily practice holding onto the end of her bed. It seemed wonderful to have a *barre* of her own, but it looked so much like hard work when Anne saw it that she made a face at it, and said, "Exercises, exercises, exercises!"

28

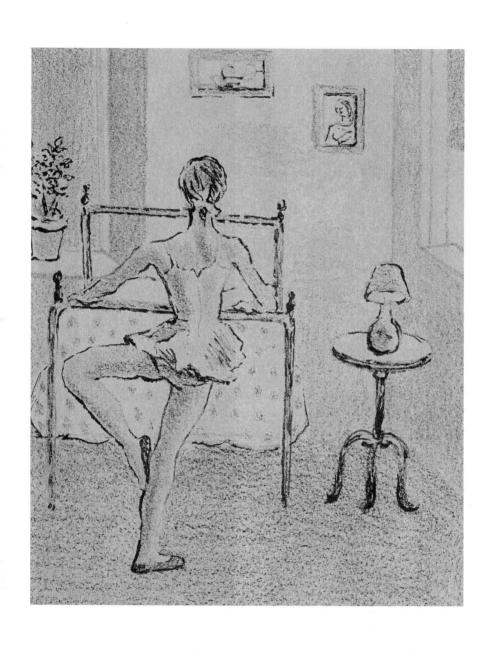

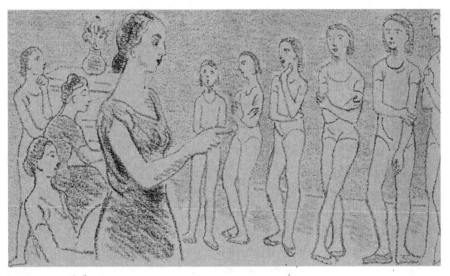

## Music

During Anne's ballet classes a pianist called Miss Alice banged out chords on the old upright piano. But Madame would not let her pupils rely on music.

"Count while you're working, girls. You won't have a piano at home," she warned. Anne tore her mind in half remembering her placing, and counting at the same time, "One and two and . . ." Every once in a while Madame would call the girls over to the piano after the lesson was over, and would ask Miss Alice to play excerpts from a ballet. Then it was surprising what music Miss Alice could get out of those battered old keys. It was surprising too how well Anne came to know ballet music.

Miss Alice would play a few measures from different ballets, the "Dance of the Swans" music by Tschaikowsky from *Swan Lake*, or perhaps a little of one of the fairy dances from *The Sleeping Princess*. Then Madame would touch first one of her pupils, then another, and tell her to mark the beat with her feet. Anne thought marking the beat was quite easy, but some of the girls found it difficult. They would lose time, and hurry to catch up, and occasionally trip over their feet.

Sometimes Madame stood the girls in a line. Then Miss Alice would play two or three measures of a well-known piece of music. It might be ballet music, or it might not, but she never chose parts that were easy to recognize. In the order in which they were standing, each girl in turn had to name the piece of music and tell who wrote it. Any girl who could not answer had to move to the foot of the line. Anne thought this game was fun. She was one of the best at it in the class.

Madame wrote to Father and Mother and asked if it were possible for Anne to take piano lessons. She said music was a very important part of dancing, and that Anne had a good ear. It would be very helpful for her to have some extra training. Though Anne had no idea of it, her music lessons meant that Father and Mother had to do without other things. Still, piano lessons were managed, and while Anne did not care for them very much, she found they helped her dancing.

31

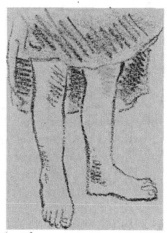

## The Third Hurdle

Toward the end of the first year, Anne began to worry. Not all the girls she had started with were still in her class, although new ones had taken the place of those who dropped out. Soon Madame would have to decide whether to go on teaching her. Did she think Anne showed promise? For what seemed a long time Anne heard nothing from Madame. Then something terrible happened. She began to have trouble with her feet.

Suddenly, without warning, they started "rolling." Everyone at school understood what rolling was, but it was Father who helped stop it. Anne came home swollen-faced and red-eyed. "My feet are rolling," she said. "Madame says if they don't get right I will have to stop taking ballet lessons!"

Father told Anne crying would not help, she was to take off

32

her shoes and socks and show him what the trouble was. But Anne could not tell what her feet were doing that was wrong. Father watched Anne's bare feet and soon saw.

"Madame means that you're using the insides of your feet, turning them so the arches are almost on the ground," he explained. After that, Father got up early for a couple of weeks to watch Anne practice. He rubbed blue chalk on the insides of both arches, and fastened white paper to the floor for her to dance on so she could tell when she turned her feet in. Thanks to Father's watchful eye and the blue chalk, Anne's feet stopped rolling, and never rolled again.

Looking back over the first year, Anne could not see that she had learned much except how to keep her feet from rolling. She did know how to feel tall, and she knew a great many exercises, as well as their correct French names. But did Madame think she was worth training?

The answer came unexpectedly at the end of a lesson. Anne stepped forward to make her *révérence*, and Madame stopped her.

"Come here, my child," she said. "Please tell your parents I shall continue to teach you. Ask your Mother to come and see me, for we have to plan your days. Next term you will begin real work."

Anne thought, "Real work! Goodness, haven't I been doing real work?" But she said only, "Thank you, Madame."

33

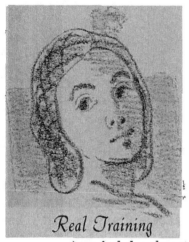

## Real Training

Anne had thought privately that the second year could not be very different from the first. But she was quite wrong. She had had three lessons a week during the first year. Now, in her second year, she had a lesson a day, and they were much longer. In the first year Anne and the other girls had sat down on the floor to rest between exercises. In the second year Madame made a rule: "Never sit during a class." There were still exercises, exercises, exercises, with Miss Alice thumping on the piano, and Madame poking with her stick as the girls practiced. But there were great changes in the way the exercises were done, and soon there were many new ones to learn.

Although she used them very little at first, Anne was told to buy blocked ballet shoes. She was terribly proud of those first ballet shoes, but she quickly found that they were not as glamorous

34

as she had thought. Box-toed, reinforced toe shoes needed break-ing-in, and breaking-in was hard work, and cruel to the feet. Her toes had to be bandaged so that they would not get bruised and bleed through to her shoes. Even though they were used until they wore out, ballet shoes would not last long and cost a lot of money. The studio floor was slippery although it was not very clean, and so every pair of ballet shoes had to be darned on the toes in order to grip the floor.

Anne found that she could not dance if her ballet shoes did not fit well and were not fastened on properly. Madame showed the class how to sew a loop to the back of the heel, and ribbons on either side of the instep. These were passed through the loop and tied securely around the ankles.

In her first year Anne had tied her hair back with two bows to keep it off her neck. Now that she was in real training Madame made her wear a net, kept in place with ribbons. Nothing, Madame said, must hide any part of a pupil. She must be able to see every bone and every muscle.

Madame liked her pupils to wear white tunics and pink tights, although the more usual dress was a leotard and tights.

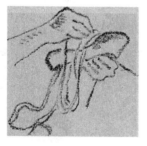

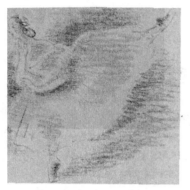

## Port de Bras

Even the most ambitious dancers have moments during their training when they almost give up. There are times when they make no progress, and even times when they seem to be going backward. Anne had very bad spells in her second year of real work. One of her great troubles was her arms.

When Anne had seen her first ballet, she had wondered how the dancers' arms could flow so smoothly. As her training went on she stopped wondering about this, for she knew the answer. Every exercise had a proper position for the arms. The arms take these positions in a continuous movement called *port de bras* (POR-duh-BRAH). The eyes and head must follow the movements of the hands.

Madame said fingers should be soft as thistledown and curved like the petals of a rose. In her first years, Anne's fingers felt like bananas and looked like them. Madame said that dancers did not have elbows, but soft curves where other people's elbows were. Anne was so conscious of her elbows that they often seemed to her not only to stick out, but to be so sharp they could cut something. Every day a teacher's voice was raised in anguish: "Anne, your arms!" Every day there were special exercises just for the arms. Miss Alice played chords, and arms were raised to the waist, softly above the head, then to the sides. The wrists were turned, and the arms brought down to the positions in which they started.

"Oh, goodness," moaned Anne, "it looks easy, it should be easy, but my arms will never learn!" Although Anne did not know it, her arms were learning, and from angular little sticks were becoming soft and flowing just as Madame said they should be.

Here are some of the arm positions Anne learned:

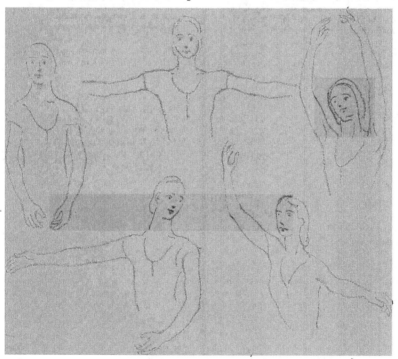

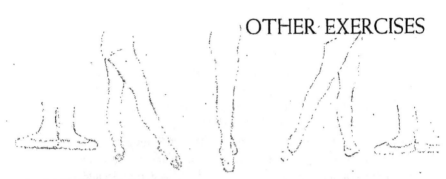

*Ronds de Jambe* (RON duh ZHAM)

These are half circles drawn with one leg while standing on the supporting leg. Starting from first position, the working foot slides forward and points straight out, then swings outward and around until the toe points back. Then the feet return to first position. In this exercise, only the working leg must move, and the knee must never bend.

*Relevé* (ruh-luh-VAY)

This means "rising." Starting from second position, facing the *barre*, the dancer jumps onto the balls of her feet, tightening her legs, then springs back into second position.

*Echappé* (ay-shap-PAY)

This is done facing the *barre*, holding onto it with both hands. The feet are in fifth position, *demi-plié*. Then there is a jump into second position *relevé*, and a jump back into fifth position *plié*.

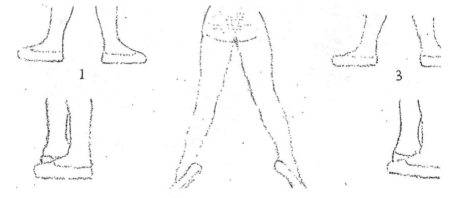

1

3

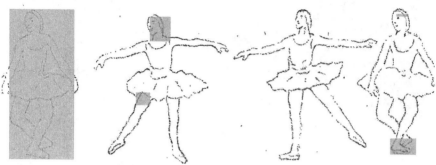

*Glissade* (glee-SAHD)

Starting with feet in fifth position, the back foot slides out through second position until it just clears the floor. The weight shifts to the foot that is out, then goes back to fifth position, *plié*. Repeat with other foot, and so on in a smooth series of motions. (See above.)

*Pas de Chat* (PAH duh SHAH)

From fifth position, the toe of the back foot is raised to the knee of the front foot. The dancer springs onto the raised foot, and lifts the toe of the other foot to that knee. For an instant both feet are off the floor. Then she returns to the fifth position *plié* and repeats the step as often as directed. (See below.)

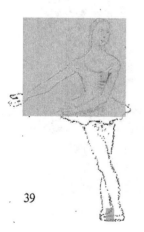

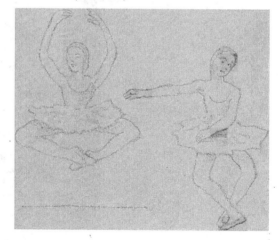

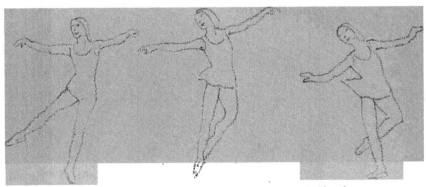

*Jeté* (zhuh-TAY)

This jump from one foot to another begins in *demi-plié*. The back foot is lifted and the knee is well turned out. The back foot goes straight out to one side, then down, and the other foot is lifted in back, slightly bent. (See above.)

*Changement de Pieds* (shanzh-MAHN duh pee-AY)

From fifth position, *demi-plié*, the dancer jumps in the air. The front foot crosses to the back while jumping, and the feet return to the ground in fifth position. (See below.)

Anne learned this first *demi-pointe*, on the balls of her feet, and later on her *pointes*, in her new satin slippers.

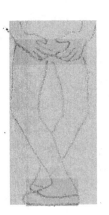

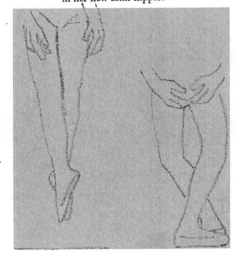

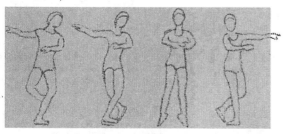 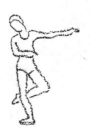

*Pas de Bourrée* (PAH duh boor-RAY)

This is perhaps the best-known step in dancing, but is very hard to describe. From fifth position *plié,* the left foot is lifted behind the right, lowered and the weight shifted onto it. The left foot goes out to second position *relevé.* Then the right leg crosses in front and the weight shifts onto it, while the left leg is lifted and bent. This is done repeatedly in a series of tiny steps. (See above.)

*Entrechat* (ahn-truh-SHAH)

This is a much harder and showier form of *changement de pieds.* It was a long time before Anne learned this step.

It begins in fifth position. The dancer jumps into the air with straight knees, and while the feet are off the ground the calves of the legs beat each other several times, forward and back. Then the feet return to the ground in fifth position. (See below.)

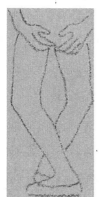 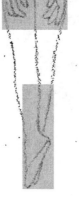 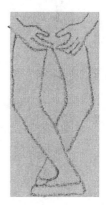

41

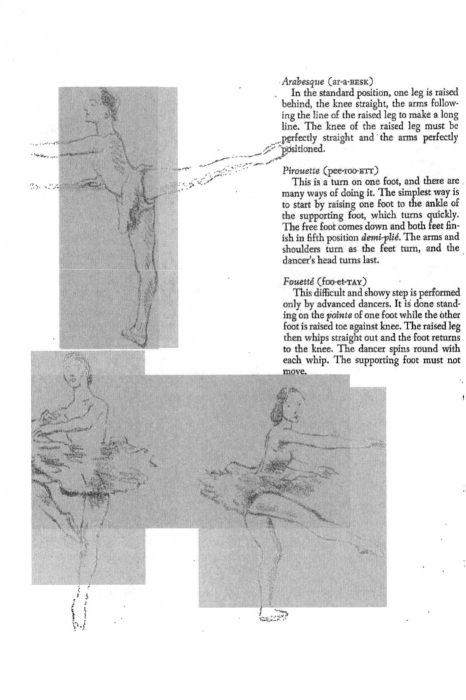

### Arabesque (ar-a-BESK)

In the standard position, one leg is raised behind, the knee straight, the arms following the line of the raised leg to make a long line. The knee of the raised leg must be perfectly straight and the arms perfectly positioned.

### Pirouette (pee-roo-ETT)

This is a turn on one foot, and there are many ways of doing it. The simplest way is to start by raising one foot to the ankle of the supporting foot, which turns quickly. The free foot comes down and both feet finish in fifth position *demi-plié*. The arms and shoulders turn as the feet turn, and the dancer's head turns last.

### Fouetté (foo-et-TAY)

This difficult and showy step is performed only by advanced dancers. It is done standing on the *pointe* of one foot while the other foot is raised toe against knee. The raised leg then whips straight out and the foot returns to the knee. The dancer spins round with each whip. The supporting foot must not move.

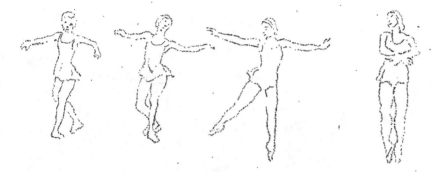

## Putting Steps Together

As Anne progressed in her dancing, center practice included *enchaînement* (ahn-shen-MAHN). This means putting a series of steps together as you use words to make a sentence. At first the *enchaînements* were short, because the girls were just learning how to remember a series of steps. But as Anne's training went on, they grew longer and longer. Learning a number of steps in order is very important to a dancer.

Anne learned many other steps, many other dancing words, and countless difficult combinations of steps. Each day she studied something new, and each day she understood more what dancing meant. She learned to use any moment of free time during a class to lie on her back with her feet propped against the wall. She learned how to keep stinging sweat out of her eyes. She learned to relax by bending so that her head was on a level with her knees. She learned the prime rule of a dancer's life: Absolutely *never* miss daily practice.

43

# THE STORY OF THE BALLET

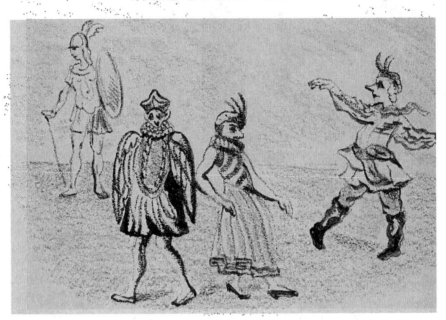

Madame taught her pupils a little of the history of the ballet. The story began four hundred years ago. It started with a young Italian girl called Catherine de Medici.

The ballets Catherine de Medici watched as a child four hundred years ago in Italy would look funny today. Only men danced, and they wore stiff clothes and high boots, so their ballet had to be a very dignified kind of dancing. But as slow, sedate and boring as it would seem to us, Catherine loved it.

When Catherine grew up she married Henry II of France. She was a very powerful queen, and when she said, "I want dancers. Send them from Italy," from Italy they came. Catherine never dreamed this meant that for the next two hundred years France would be the true home of ballet. Nor could she have guessed that someday, because of her, young dancers all over the world would have to learn the French words for every exercise and step they studied. (Even the word "ballet" is French, from the Italian word *balletto* meaning "a little dance.")

Catherine had been dead over fifty years when Louis XIV came to the throne of France. Louis XIV was extremely fond of ballet.

He had a new idea. He wanted *girls* to dance in the court ballets, too. He established the first French Academy of Dancing and gave orders that girls were to be accepted as pupils.

When the Academy's pupils were trained, they gave public performances. Now for the first time ordinary people outside court circles were able to see ballets. Soon the news spread throughout Europe, and other countries asked the Academy to supply trained dancers as teachers. The Academy sent dancers all over Europe.

The girls who had learned dancing at the Academy of Louis XIV wore heavy clothes, tight, boned bodices, and skirts right down to the ground. A dancer called Marie Camargo, who lived in the

45

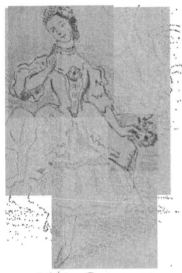

*Marie Camargo*

middle of the eighteenth century, changed the style of dress, and in doing so made ballet more like the dancing we know now. She dared to have her skirts cut short enough to show her ankles, and had the heels taken off her shoes. Her clothes caused a sensation! For the first time the audience could see exactly what the dancer's feet and ankles were doing. Of course, Camargo was also able to move much more freely than dancers had done before. It is almost certain that she danced at least some of the basic steps that are used today.

A hundred years later came a dancer named Marie Taglioni. She was a new sort of dancer altogether. She danced with ease and grace and always made sure she was well placed. Taglioni was one of the very few dancers who could leap into the air and pause before she came down. Her balance was perfect. Most interesting of all, she was the first ballerina who really danced beautifully on the tips of her toes.

Many lovely romantic ballets were created for Taglioni, which she danced in full, gauzy skirts. She went to Russia, and was a great success there.

Ten years after Taglioni first danced in St. Petersburg, a man joined the company who was to have an important influence on ballet. He was a Frenchman named Marius Petipa. First he was a dancer, but some years later he was appointed ballet master, and taught and rehearsed the dancers of the company.

Until Taglioni appeared, dancing had been largely posturing and gesturing, and beauty of movement and line had not been important. Petipa taught Taglioni's kind of dancing and improved on it. He invented a technique of ballet

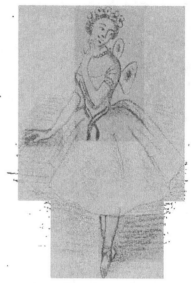

*Marie Taglioni*

which all his pupils had to study. (The young men, of course, were given a completely different kind of training from the girls, just as they are today.)

Petipa sent to Italy for dancers who were famous for a showy technique which included great leaps and difficult steps. Among them was a ballerina named Pierrina Legnani, who was the first dancer to do thirty-two *fouettés*. Oddly enough, Petipa never really approved of the Italian acrobatic dancing. He thought nothing was more beautiful than the stylized French dancing which he had helped perfect.

47

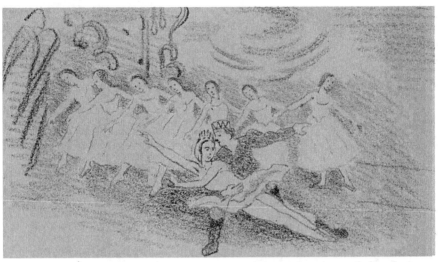

Petipa was a ballet master of the Imperial Russian Ballet for fifty years. He introduced many of the steps and arm movements that are taught today, and gave us some of our most famous ballets, such as *Swan Lake*.

Long after the first visit of the impressive Italian dancers, an Italian named Enrico Cecchetti was engaged as ballet master of another company of the Imperial Russian Ballet. The rivalry between his school of dancing and Petipa's seemed to bring out the finest qualities of both kinds of ballet. The combination of Italian technique and French grace and elegance produced the classic, or Russian, style of ballet. The Russian ballet dancers cut their dresses very short in order not to hide anything of the precision of their movements.

By the early years of the twentieth century, Marius Petipa was an old man. To many of the new dancers, his methods of teaching and theory of what ballet should be seemed too rigid. The feeling of being repressed was strong in Michel Fokine, a young dancer of great ability.

Fokine was not only a fine dancer but also a wonderful creator of ballets. He thought that the ballet had become too set in its ways. Another man, Serge Diaghilev, was thinking the same sort of thing at this time. Diaghilev was not a dancer, a choreographer (kor-ee-OG-ra-fer)—a person who arranges dance steps into a pattern—or a musician. He was just a ballet-lover. He formed an

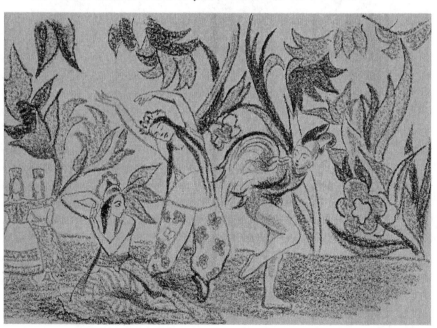

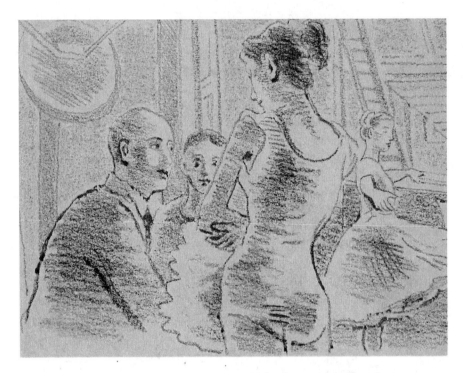

outstandingly talented company of Russian dancers, musicians, stage designers and choreographers and took them to Europe. Among them were Fokine and a dancer of great artistry named Anna Pavlova.

Until Diaghilev formed his ballet troupe, no one had thought of creating a ballet as a combined operation. Choreographers had worked alone, finding stories and arranging steps that would tell

50

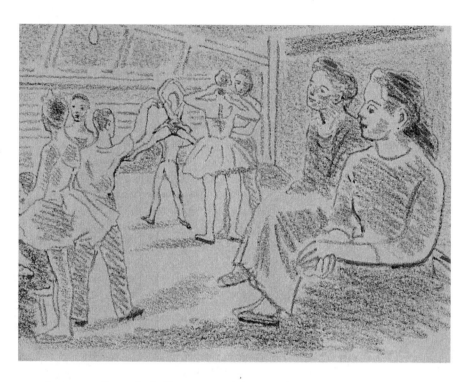

the stories. Once the ballet was in production, costume and scenery designers had set to work. They knew what the ballet was about, but they had never thought of discussing their plans with the choreographer. When the dancers had started to learn their parts, they had often asked permission to leave out steps and movements that did not show them off to advantage. Sometimes they were allowed instead to put in a sequence of steps from another ballet.

But Diaghilev saw his company as a little world in which everyone contributed his or her talent to a final glowing result. And he brought out superb ballets such as *The Three-Cornered Hat* and *Prince Igor.*

Diaghilev engaged Enrico Cecchetti to teach his dancers. Under his guidance their dancing was a miracle of perfection, and the ballets were performed exactly as they were planned by the choreographer.

Perhaps the most perfect ballet of the Diaghilev company was *Petrouchka,* about puppets that come to life. It is a wonderful example of pooled talents. Igor Stravinsky, the composer, and Alexander Benois, a stage designer, thought of the story. Michel Fokine did the choreography. Stravinsky wrote the music for it, and Benois designed the scenery and costumes. One of the greatest male dancers who ever lived danced *Petrouchka:* Vaslav Nijinsky. Like Taglioni, he was able to pause in the air in the middle of a leap before coming to the ground.

The conferences between all those concerned in the production of the Diaghilev ballets brought about not only wonderful dancing, music and choreography, but also rich, vivid colors and striking new designs in the scenery and costumes. Except in certain ballets, gone were the old formal ballet dresses and wreaths of flowers. Ever since Diaghilev's time, nothing surprises us in the design and costuming of a ballet.

52

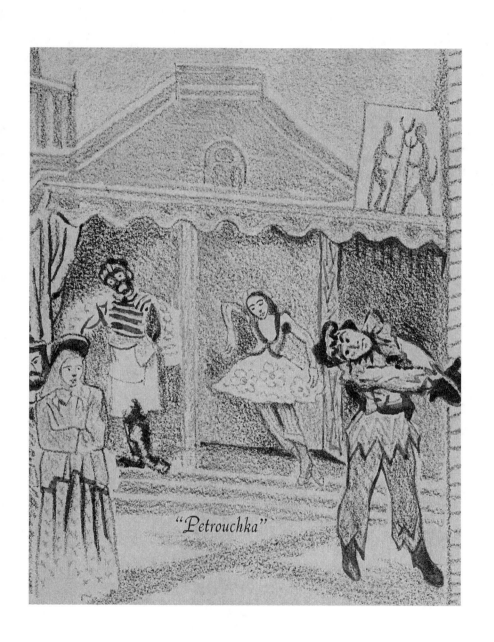

"*Petrouchka*"

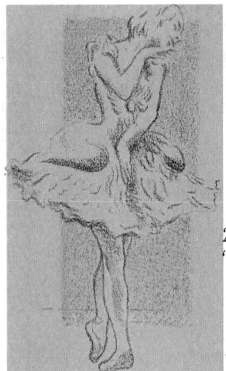

*Anna Pavlova in
"The Dying Swan"*

Anna Pavlova did not dance very long with the Diaghilev company, but formed her own troupe after a time. Her most famous dance was written for her by Fokine to music by Saint-Saëns. It was called *The Dying Swan*. She chose and trained herself a group of young girls, and with them toured the world. Wherever she went she lit flames in people's hearts. To those who

had never before known about the ballet, the beauty of her dancing came as something new. They began to think of ballet dancing
as a serious career for young girls and boys, and ballet schools
sprang up wherever Pavlova had danced.

A great personality who first became known in Diaghilev's
company is Leonide Massine. Massine is both a fine dancer and
a fine choreographer. His work forms a link between modern ballet and the classic style of the Imperial Russian Ballet.

For a while after Diaghilev's death in 1929, it seemed to ballet lovers that ballet had died too. But of course it had not. There
were people who continued the tradition.

The first ballet company to arise after Diaghilev's company
broke up was the Ballet Russe de Monte Carlo, formed by Colonel
de Basil and René Blum of the French ballet. They performed
the ballets Diaghilev's dancers had made famous, and had successful seasons in England, in Europe and in the United States.

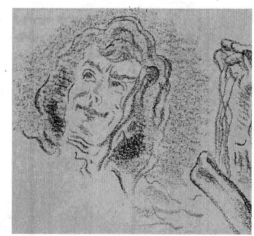

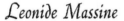

*Leonide Massine*

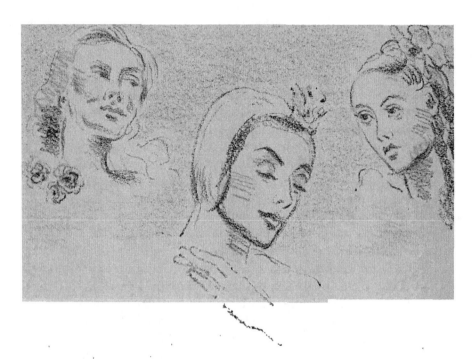

Three very young girls were the chief performers of the Ballet
Russe de Monte Carlo: Irina Baronova, Tamara Toumanova, and
Tatiana Riabouchinska. All of them were under fifteen when they
became stars. People flocked to see them as well as Alexandra
Danilova, a famous ballerina who joined the company later. An-
other great dancer and choreographer who went to the Ballet
Russe de Monte Carlo was Georges Balanchine. He retained and
revived the beauty of the classic ballets.

In the meantime other people were working quietly, and after a time their efforts bore fruit. A woman named Ninette de Valois founded a ballet group called the Camargo Society in London and, years later, the famous Sadler's Wells Ballet Company. In London, too, Marie Rambert started a small experimental group at the Mercury Theater. She has discovered many talented dancers and choreographers over the years, among them such famous ones as Frederick Ashton and Anthony Tudor.

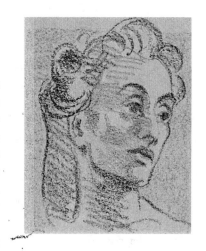

*Ninette de Valois*

In France ballet continued to prosper in association with the Paris Opera. The Russian State Ballet was flourishing, but it did not inspire or help other ballet companies because so few outsiders have been able to see anything of the Russian dancers since the Revolution. In America it took a long time for successful ballet companies to be born, but once they were, ballet took vigorous root.

The Ballet Russe de Monte Carlo came to the United States in 1933 and found its programs very popular. Most of them were based on the exciting ballets the Diaghilev company had created, but several times "American" ballets were attempted. They did not last, however, and it was not until after native ballet companies had been established that Agnes de Mille choreographed a really fine American ballet for the Ballet Russe: *Rodeo.*

One of the most outstanding American troupes was the Ballet Theater Company, founded in 1939 by a woman named Lucia Chase. She perhaps more than anyone else helped American ballet come into its own. She introduced not only Americans dancing the great classic ballets, but also choreography of a new kind, free and expressive, and truly American. Two great American choreographers worked for the Ballet Theater: Jerome Robbins, who created *Fancy Free,* and Agnes de Mille, who created *Fall River Legend.* Agnes de Mille believes in flawless technique, but she has "twisted" the technique so that classically trained dancers can perform folk steps. More than that, it was she who brought about the change in musical-comedy shows from the traditional chorus of pretty girls without talent to imaginative dancing by well-trained performers. Ever since the success of her ballet scenes in *Oklahoma,* almost every musical show has had really fine dancing. Today musicals need a large number of first-class dancers to draw upon, and be-

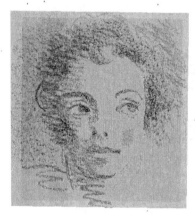

*Agnes de Mille*

58

cause of this the general standard of training has improved.

Georges Balanchine stayed only a short time with the de Basil company, and has been connected with American ballet for many years. He was the founder of the New York City Ballet, and became one of its great choreographers. He married the internationally famous ballerina Maria Tallchief.

Today there is an increasing use of ballet in movies: *Red Shoes, An American in Paris,* and *Hans Christian Andersen* are among the finest.

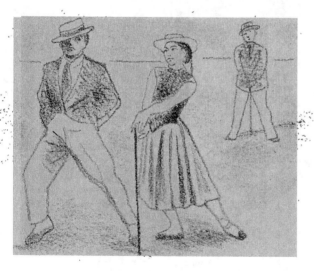

*Leslie Caron in "An American in Paris"*

# WELL-KNOWN BALLERINAS

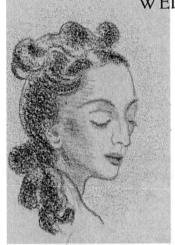

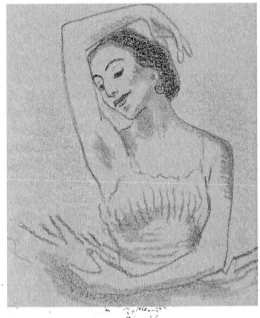

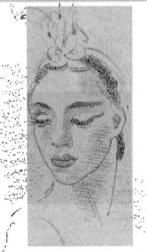

*Reading clockwise:*

ALEXANDRA DANILOVA studied at the Imperial Russian School of Ballet before the Revolution and was a star in the Soviet State Ballet Company. Now she is a *prima ballerina* with the Ballet Russe de Monte Carlo.

ALICIA MARKOVA, an English girl, started with the Diaghilev ballet troupe. She danced with early English ballet companies, and when she left the Sadler's Wells Ballet she formed her own company with choreographer Anton Dolin. Since World War II she has danced in America almost exclusively.

MARIA TALLCHIEF, of American Indian descent, trained with Bronislava Nijinska, Vaslav Nijinsky's sister, and other fine teachers. She is especially noted for her beautiful dancing of classic roles.

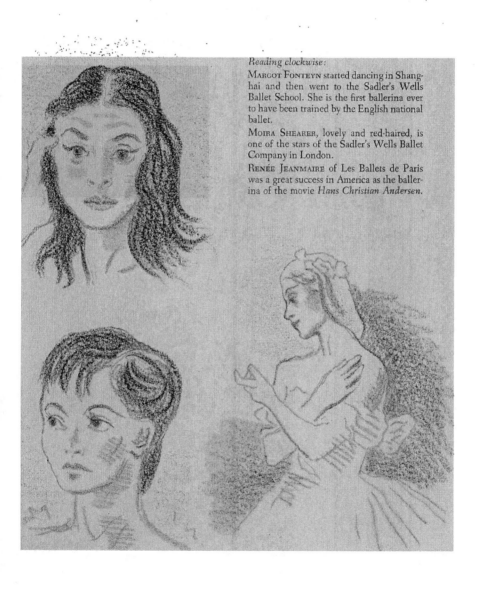

*Reading clockwise:*

MARGOT FONTEYN started dancing in Shanghai and then went to the Sadler's Wells Ballet School. She is the first ballerina ever to have been trained by the English national ballet.

MOIRA SHEARER, lovely and red-haired, is one of the stars of the Sadler's Wells Ballet Company in London.

RENÉE JEANMAIRE of Les Ballets de Paris was a great success in America as the ballerina of the movie *Hans Christian Andersen.*

# FAMOUS BALLETS

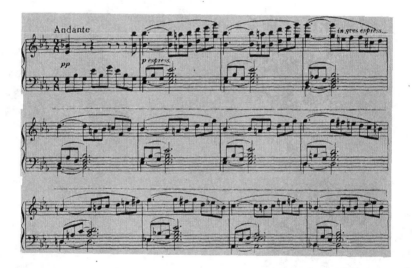

GISELLE is a romantic ballet in two acts. It tells the story of a peasant girl who died when she discovered that her lover had to marry a princess. A girl who dies before her wedding day is supposed to become a kind of ghost. The ghosts come out of their graves at night and dance till dawn. As Giselle dances in the churchyard where she is buried, her lover sees her, dances with her, and dies on her grave.

This is the oldest ballet that has come down to us in its exact form.

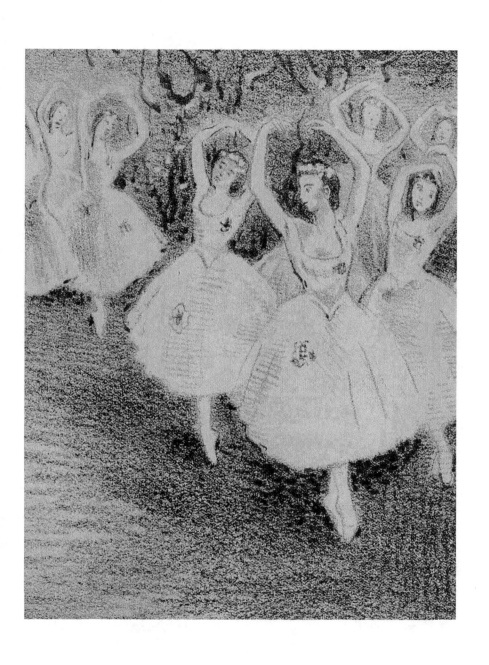

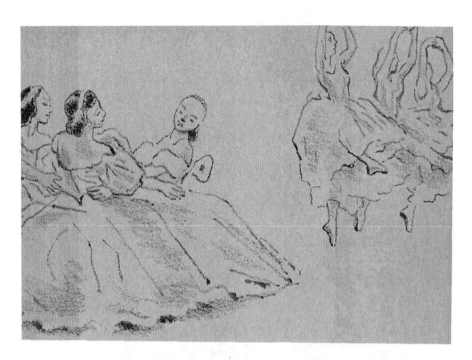

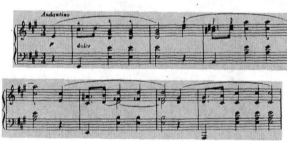

LES SYLPHIDES (lay sil-FEED) is a ballet in the romantic manner created by Michel Fokine. It does not tell a story, but creates a mood, in which the spirits of the wood dance in a forest to music by Chopin.

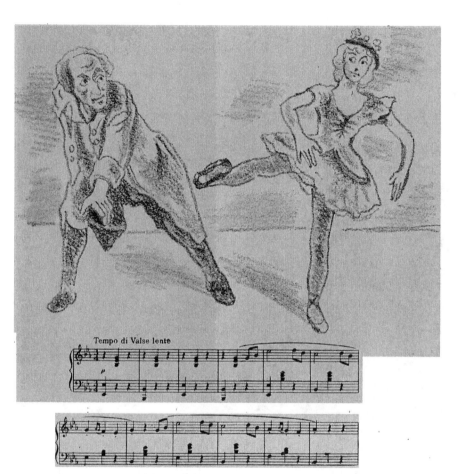

Tempo di Valse lente

COPPELIA, a classic ballet, is about a doll and a girl named Swanhilda. Swanhilda does not know that Coppelia is a doll and grows jealous of her, because she thinks her fiancé, Frantz, is falling in love with Coppelia. Swanhilda gets into the workshop of the old toymaker who created Coppelia, changes clothes with the doll, and fools the old man into thinking Coppelia has come alive. Frantz comes to see what is going on. After it is all explained he and Swanhilda get married. The old toymaker is given a bag of gold.

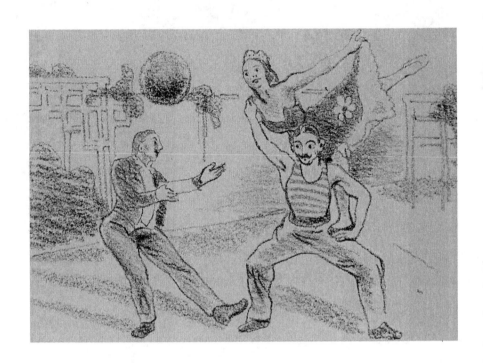

LE BEAU DANUBE (luh boh dan-yoon) is a ballet by Massine, based
on music by Johann Strauss. It is a gay, funny modern ballet set in old
Vienna, in which all the characters are dressed in different shades of brown.
It takes place in a park on a public holiday.

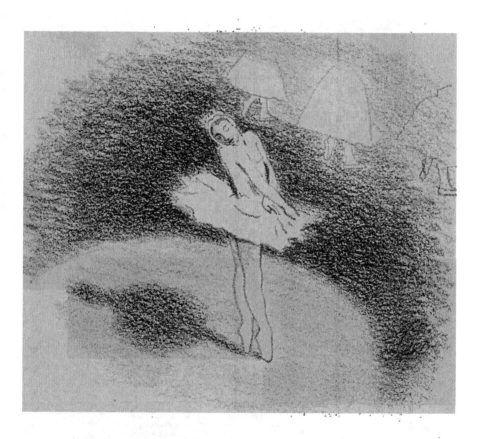

SWAN LAKE is a classic ballet by Petipa set to music by Tschaikowsky. It is about a girl named Odette whom a sorcerer has turned into a swan. She and the other swans glide across a lake in the forest one moonlit night, and a prince who is out hunting tries to shoot them. But Odette becomes a human girl at midnight, and the prince falls in love with her. He invites her to come to a ball at which he is to choose his bride. Odette says she cannot do so and the prince is heartbroken.

In the end the sorcerer's spell is broken because the prince is willing to die for Odette. All the swans regain their human form.

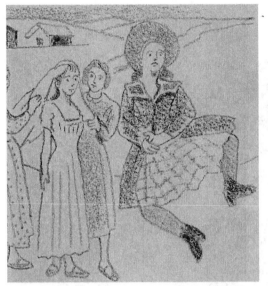

## OKLAHOMA

One part of the famous musical show is a modern ballet called "Laurie Makes Up Her Mind." In it the heroine, who wonders whether she should marry a boy named Curley, falls asleep and dreams about her wedding.

## PETER AND THE WOLF

is a modern ballet which has music by Prokofieff. It tells about a little boy, Peter, and his friends the duck, the bird and the cat, who go into the forest. The wolf runs off with the duck, but Peter captures him. In the end hunters help Peter bring the wolf to the zoo.

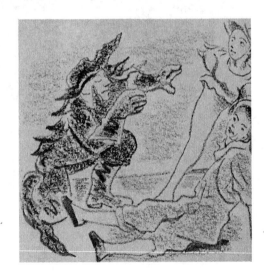

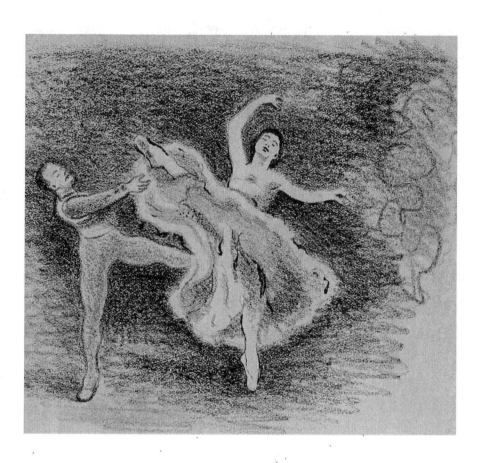

JARDIN AUX LILAS (zhar-DAN oh lee-LAH),which means Lilac Garden,
is a modern ballet by Anthony Tudor. It tells the story of a girl named Caro-
line, who is going to be married, and her fiancé. They both have had other
sweethearts whom they hate to leave, and as the couples dance their feelings
are clearly shown.

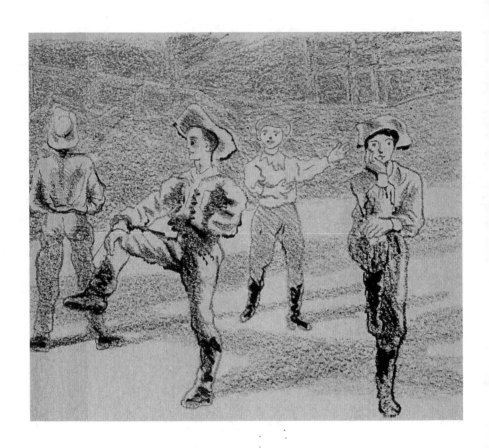

RODEO, a modern American ballet by Agnes de Mille, is about a cowgirl who tries to be as bold and clever as the cowboys. She goes to a party dressed in her usual clothes, and no one will dance with her until she changes into a party dress. When she does, she is the most attractive girl there.

## Back to the Family

Anne discovered that everything Madame had said about the difficulty of training to be a dancer was true. Equally true was what she had said about the way dancing would eat up her leisure. As month followed month, Anne felt herself being pulled further away from ordinary family life into the dancer's world.

Father and Mother watched Anne slipping away from the family, and Father decided at last that he must put a stop to it.

"Anne," he said one day, "it's over two years now that you've been having ballet lessons. You're doing very well, and Mother and I are proud of you, but we don't want to lose our daughter. These last few months you come home in a dream, go to bed in a dream, get up in a dream. We'd like to have some of your company for a change."

Anne thought this over and saw what Father meant. She tried to explain to him what had happened.

"I have so many lessons I don't get much time to think, and a lot of dancing is thinking. Then, too, when we come to classes Madame likes us to feel sort of ballet-ish—to be full of nothing but dancing. It means I have to stop being the real Anne when I go to the studio, and be Anne again only when I leave it. I think I've got into the habit of being dancing Anne all the time now, if you know what I mean."

Father said he knew just what she meant, and that was what he and Mother did not like. It would be nice if sometimes their own Anne, and not dancing Anne, came home in the evenings. How would it be if she gave the twins dancing lessons?

Anne shuddered at the idea, but tried it anyway, and the lessons were an enormous success with the whole family. The twins were nearly as round as they were tall. Neither could tell her left foot from her right one. Anne started them with the five positions, and the arm movements that went with them. The house rang with laughter at their efforts. Then Anne tried to teach the twins half bends. Before long Mother was doing half bends as she cooked, and Father, half bends as he shaved in the morning. Even though the twins had no talent, teaching them did Anne a lot of good, for she took herself and her dancing less seriously. After all, a dancing career was still just a possibility for her. It was foolish to live, eat and sleep nothing but ballet. Keeping on as she had been would make her grow up one-sided, and it would be hard for her if a dancing career turned out impossible.

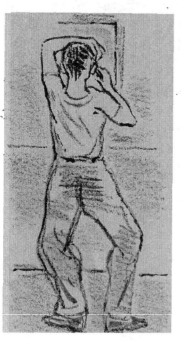

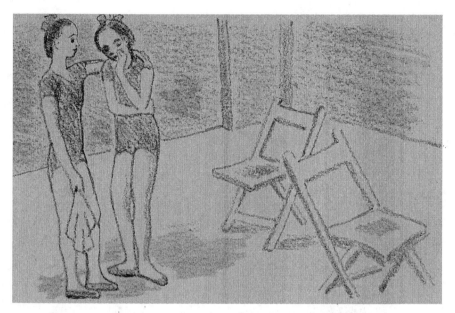

It was two or three months after Father had pulled Anne back into the family that she understood how wise he had been. So far all the girls who had started serious training with Anne had gone right along with her. Now a girl called Mary left. Mary had always been the slowest of the group. She was not built well for a dancer. Mary had short legs and arms, a long body and rather stiff feet. One day Anne had come back after class to get some clothes she had left behind. Suddenly she saw Mary, alone, holding onto the *barre* and sobbing.

"I can't bear it! I can't. I won't bear it. I *must* be a dancer, there's nothing else I care about or can do!"

At first Anne thought she would go out softly and pretend she had not heard. Then that seemed mean. She came over to Mary and put an arm round her. "Won't Madame teach you any more?" Anne asked.

Mary kept on sobbing, but soon the story poured out. Madame had been nice, so nice she couldn't have been nicer, but she said she saw no future in dancing for Mary. "Madame says my Achilles tendon doesn't stretch properly, and she doesn't think it ever will. But it isn't only that . . . ." and Mary cried louder, "she says in the last months she has watched me carefully and I've grown worse! I've gone backwards."

Anne asked sympathetically, "Isn't there any other kind of dancing you could do? You don't need our kind of training for all dancing."

Mary said, "That's what I thought, but Madame says that the trend is to use ballet-trained dancers for all good dancing. And I know I wouldn't have a chance in a musical unless I was a marvelous dancer, because I'm not pretty, and I'm getting fat. Madame said the best thing I could do was go on with my education, and forget about dancing for the time being. She was certain that I would find I was interested in something else quite soon. Oh, I do wish I hadn't given up everything for dancing. It's so hard now that I'm not going to dance any more."

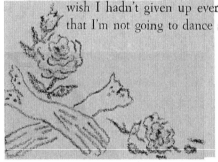

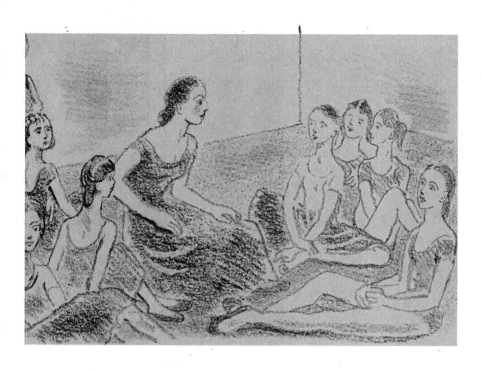

## Settling for Something Else

A few months later a girl called Helen left the school. This time the ending was happier. Madame called the whole school together and spoke to them.

"I know you were all very sorry for Mary, but you have been warned that you would have to stop if I and my teachers did not think you would make a dancer. Later on Mary will find that she

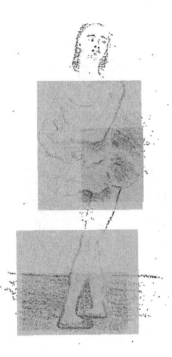

wasted no time in this school, for what she has learned about dancing here will make her enjoy watching it all her life.

"After today Helen is going away, but she is only leaving us to attend a different kind of dancing school. She has given me permission to show you why. Over and over again I and the other teachers have said to Helen, 'I don't *want* to know you are going to do a difficult step. Every step in classical ballet must melt into the next step.' Now, school, I want you to notice that Helen cannot help saying with her whole body, 'Watch me do this. See how smart I am.'. . . Helen, will you show us that *enchaînement* we worked on last week."

Miss Alice played a chord, and Helen stepped into the center of the room. Now that Madame had explained it, everybody could see what she meant. As Helen completed a step, they had to laugh, for from the top of her head to the tips of her fingers, all of her said, "There! Now clap."

Madame laughed too and put a hand on Helen's shoulder. She said Helen was going to a very famous stage dancing school, and it would not surprise her if later on Helen made quite a name for herself.

The next day Madame talked seriously to Anne's class. She said that she wanted her pupils to be able to join any great ballet company. They must all have had a thorough training, so that they could dance in any type of ballet, and this meant the great classical ballets as well as the moderns. What they had to learn was "lyricism." This meant that every movement must flow; there must never be a carefully planned start that made the audience think "Now we're going to see something."

Anne learned a great deal from what Madame said. She knew inside her what lyricism meant, and though she was afraid Madame could not see it, she thought sometimes there was a little lyricism in her own dancing.

77

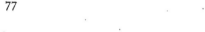

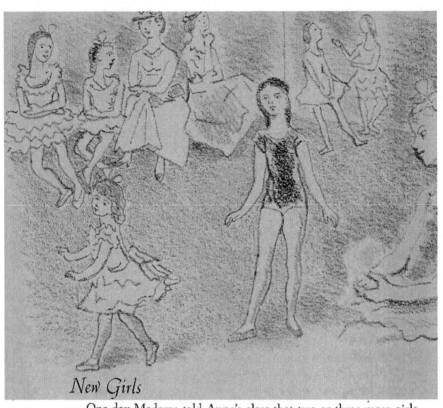

## New Girls

One day Madame told Anne's class that two or three more girls might join them. Later on in their training they would work with a class of boys who were her pupils. There were a great many lifts and steps which they would need to know when dancing with a partner. That, of course, was in the future. But she did not think four was a large enough class, since they might grow fewer.

At this the girls looked horrified, and Madame said that she hoped to go on training them all, but you never knew what was in store for you. The girls might grow too fat or too tall. Madame was holding an audition for partly trained students on Saturday. The girls could come to it if they were quiet, and they might learn something from it.

It was very hard for Anne not to laugh at the audition, because most of the girls who came to it were funny. There were three very little girls, each of them dressed in fussy *tutus*. There were eight other girls of various sizes and shapes, too. One was dressed sensibly in a leotard and woolen tights. The others wore silk or satin tunics or ballet dresses. All the girls, except the one in the leotard, had their hair hanging loose, and all of them had mothers with them.

Most of the mothers talked a great deal. They wanted to tell Madame how wonderful their daughters were, and what other people had said about them. The mother of a tiny girl in royal blue tulle said over and over again, "You just can't believe what a wonderful little dancer my Shirley is. She has stood on her toes since she was a baby. Her teacher says she's a little Pavlova!"

Madame did not seem to hear what any of the mothers said. She rapped her stick on the floor, pointed to the girl in the leotard, and said, "I will try you."

Leotard, whose name was Judith, was the only possibility. When she had watched all the girls dance, Madame spoke tactfully to the mothers. They all left after that. Then a strange thing happened. The door flew open and a small plain girl in a crushed ballet dress came back and ran up to Madame. She looked scared but determined.

"I go to a dreadful school. I *know* I'm learning all wrong," she said. "I didn't want to wear this terrible dress. They made me do it. But I know I can dance, truly I can, if only you will give me a chance. Please teach me!"

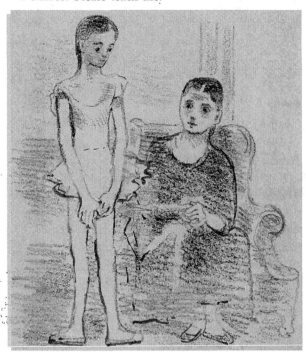

Madame thought in silence for a long time. Then she said: "Come back on Monday with your hair in a net, and wearing a bathing suit or anything else that won't hide your body, and I shall examine your feet. If your feet have not been ruined and I think you show promise, I might give you a chance. But you would have to start with the beginners. You would not only have a great deal to learn to catch up with girls of your own age, but a great deal to unlearn. Are you prepared for such hard work?"

The girl, whose name was Elizabeth, looked as if Madame had given her a handful of jewels. She made quite a nice *révérence* and said, "Thank you. You'll never be sorry."

Judith was put in Anne's class and in no time was up to the standard of the others, but months went by before Elizabeth joined them. When she did she surprised the other girls. There was something about her dancing which made it stand out. But only Madame and Elizabeth knew what catching up had cost. Madame knew of the hours of work that must have gone on at home to get her positioning right. She knew how often Elizabeth stayed behind for private lessons. She guessed how many tears of despair Elizabeth had shed, and how many sweat-soaked towels and socks Elizabeth had taken home at the end of lessons. Sometimes Madame gave Elizabeth a few of her rare words of praise. More often than the other girls, Elizabeth heard, "Well done, my child."

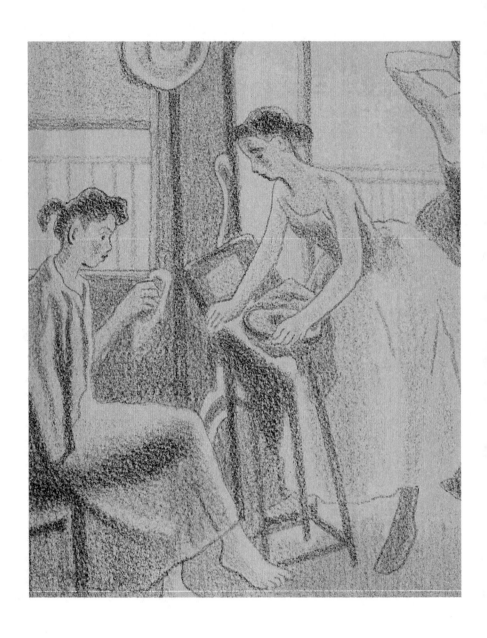

## Choreography

When a new ballet company visited the town, Madame said it was time Anne's class knew something about choreography.

"Most people imagine a ballet is written down in a book," she told them. "This dancer enters here, the following steps take her to here, the *corps de ballet* come in here. They perform the following steps which take them to here.

"But until now ballets have never been written down. The steps of the old ballets are known just as folk dances are known, because they have been taught by one generation to another. Just as in folk dancing, it is not the person who composed the dance who teaches the next generation, but the person who danced it.

"Ballets have been handed down from one trained dancer to another. Dancers remember steps partly by listening to the music, but also they remember with their muscles. Many times a dancer has been asked at short notice to take part in a ballet that she has danced, perhaps, only once before. What happens is that as the music is played, step by step her muscles remind her what her body should do."

She went on, "It was not so difficult to remember exactly what the choreographer had intended in the old classic and romantic ballets. Then when a certain step was performed, each part of the

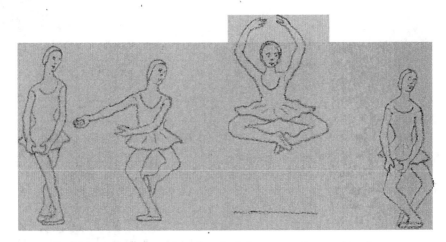

body was to do exactly what had been taught in the classrooms of the past."

To show them what she meant, Madame said, take a *pas de chat*. "The hands are down in front when you start. They are raised as you lift your foot to jump. They are raised higher as you land on the foot you are jumping on. As you complete the step, the wrists turn and the hands drop to where they started. When a *pas de chat* was danced in the old ballets, that was what the arms were doing. Nowadays nothing is certain. Modern choreographers go to a great deal of trouble to change the traditional movements. The movements they want are very often the opposite of what has been learned in the classroom.

"There is a great deal of pantomime in modern ballets, too.

84

You attend special classes to learn to express with your faces and your bodies all kinds of emotions, and to make yourselves like different types of people. But it is not something you can explain in words."

Only a descriptive phrase or two can be written, she said: "The old man looks very cross," or "a young girl dances, rejoicing in the spring." But the words don't tell the dancer *how* the old man looked cross, or in what way the young girl shows her joy in the spring.

Madame went to a blackboard and drew several patterns of curving lines.

"Here are some of the plans for the ballet *Symphonie Concer-tante*, for which Georges Balanchine did the choreography," she said. "You can see where the girls stand at the beginning, and

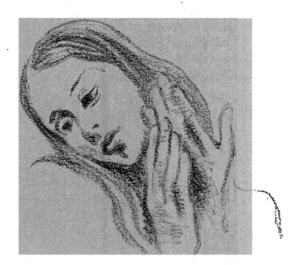

how the principal dancers cross. You can see that *Symphonie Concertante*, like all other ballets, is a series of designs. Given the plans for a ballet, any trained dancer could see the shape it ought to be if the music for it were played. But she could not tell what steps were to be danced, what arm movements used or what expressions should appear on the faces. The further away ballets move from pure classic dancing, the more difficult it is to revive one and be sure it is danced as the choreographer intended, unless there are dancers present who have done it before. I have seen a choreographer find out that the movements he had planned for his new ballet did not work out well. I watched him feel with his feet for a step. The dancers' eyes were glued to him and, as he found it, they started to move with him. Before the choreographer realized it, that step was decided on together with the arm and head movements that went with it. The next time that part of the music was reached, the choreographer saw his half-born idea being performed again because some of the dancers remembered it. He might even have forgotten exactly what he planned, but because the dancers remembered it did not matter.

"I hope very much that my pupils will be receptive to new ideas, eager to *feel* what a choreographer wants. I should like it still more if some of my pupils created dances themselves, some-day, but that is in the lap of the gods. Choreographers are born, not taught."

86

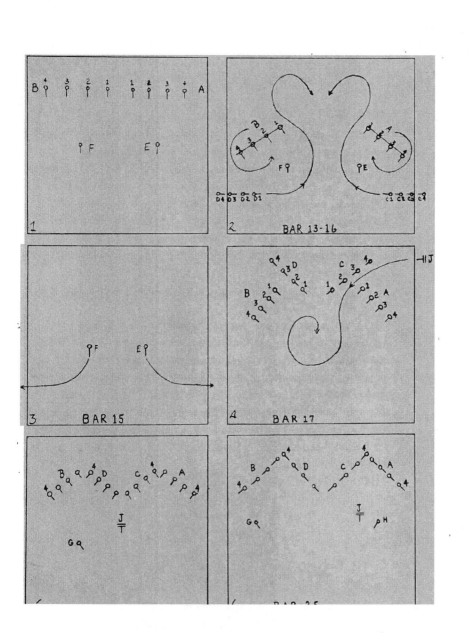

1

2    BAR 13-16

3    BAR 15

4    BAR 17

## A Dancer Is Born

. Months went by without anything special happening to Anne. Once Madame said she had good elevation, and this was important. Elevation, which meant jumping high, did not impress Madame unless it was beautifully done. Every day the girls were told there was nothing wonderful about rising high in the air, unless every part of their bodies was placed right while they were off the ground. There were times when Anne was called out to the center to dance alone and show the other girls how soft and flowing movements could be. The days when she was called out to show something to the rest of the class came more often, but they were still very far apart.

To Madame, the wise woman who would not accept a pupil unless she saw the makings of a dancer, Anne became a secret joy. Lately, there have been moments when Madame has caught her breath in sheer amazement at the beauty of some movement Anne made. Now she is beginning to make plans. When Anne is ready, she is to have her opportunity. First she will start in the *corps de ballet*, then go on to some little parts, but in the ballet company to which Madame will send her, talent is never overlooked. Anne will have her chance.

When Madame dreams she sees Anne's name in lights over a

theater. In her mind she is walking into that theater, and settling back in her seat. The music starts, and the curtain rises. The girl in the spotlight is Anne. This is the moment Madame has been working toward for many years. Now she can see the miracle. The awkward little schoolgirl, clinging to a *barre*, has turned into this exquisite fairy-like creature. A real dancer has been born.

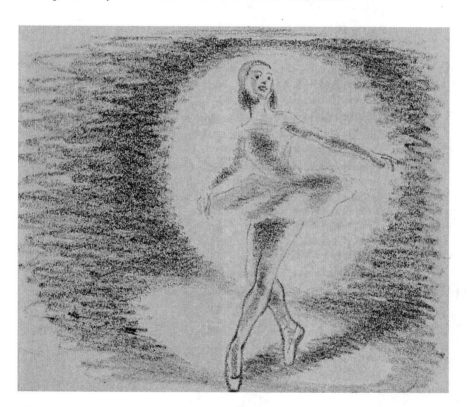

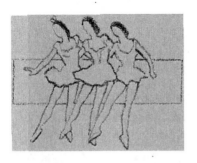

# BALLET TERMS

*arabesque* (ar-a-BESK)—A classic ballet pose which has many variations. The dancer balances on one leg and extends the other to form a long line from finger-tips to toe-tips.

*ballerina* (bal-uh-REE-na)—A female "star" ballet dancer.

*ballet* (bal-LAY)—A stylized dance which tells a story or creates a mood.

*barre* (bar)—A fixed wooden railing which dancers hold as they practice to help them balance.

*battement frappé* (bat-MAHN frap-PAY)—A small kick starting from the ankle of the supporting foot and returning to it.

*battement tendu* (bat-MAHN tahn-DU)—A small kick in which the tip of the toe slides out and remains on the floor. The knee stays straight and the leg is turned out.

*center practice*—The second half of a ballet lesson, in which the *barre* is not used for balance.

*changé* (shahn-ZHAY)—A change of feet.

*changement de pieds* (shanzh-MAHN duh pee-AY)—A small jump in which the feet change position in mid air.

90

*choreography* (kor-ee-OG-ra-fee)—The art of arranging dance steps into a pattern.

*corps de ballet* (core duh bal-LAY)—The less trained dancers in a ballet who dance only as a group.

*demi-plié* (dem-mee plee-AY)—A half bend of the knees.

*échappé* (ay-shap-PAY)—A quick movement of the feet from fifth position *plié*, jumping to second position *relevé*, ending in fifth position *plié*.

*elevation*—The height to which a dancer can jump.

*enchaînement* (ahn-shen-MAHN)—Putting dance steps together.

*entrechat* (ahn-truh-SHAH)—A jump from fifth position in which the legs beat front and back several times while in the air.

*five positions*—The first foot and arm exercises a ballet dancer learns. They are basic positions from which all movements start and in which they all end.

*fouetté* (foo-et-TAY)—A series of turns on one leg, the other leg whipping the body around.

*glissade* (glee-SAHD)—A gliding step.

*grand plié* (grahn plee-AY)—A deep knee bend.

*jeté* (zhuh-TAY)—A jump.

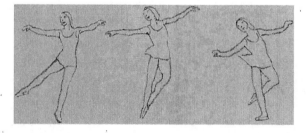

*leotard* (LEE-oh-tahrd)—A one-piece knit practice costume.

*pantomime* (PAN-tuh-mihm)—Expression by means of gestures.

*pas de bourreé* (PAH duh boor-RAY)—A series of tiny steps in which the legs seem to weave in and out.

*pas de chat* (PAH duh SHAH)—The "cat step." A light spring, something like a cat's pounce.

*petit battement* (peh-TEE bat-MAHN)—Small beats of the foot in front and in back of the ankle of the supporting leg.

*pirouette* (pee-roo-ETT)—A complete turn of the body done while standing on one leg.

*plié* (plee-AY)—A knee bend.

*pointes* (pwahnt)—Tips of the toes.

*port de bras* (POR duh BRAH)—Continuous graceful movement of the arms through a series of positions.

*relevé* (ruh-luh-VAY)—Rising up on the toes.

*révérence* (ray-vay-RAHNS)—A special bow or curtsey dancers make.

*ronds de jambe* (RON duh ZHAM)—Half circles made by the working foot while the supporting foot stands still.

*tutu* (too-TOO)—A full skirt worn by ballet dancers, usually made of many layers of thin material.

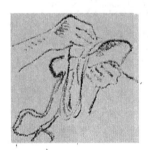

# BOOKS FOR
# BALLET-LOVERS

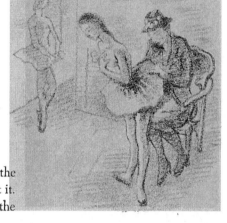

Once you've gotten interested in the ballet, you'll want to read more about it. Here are some outstanding books on the subject:

FROST, HONOR: *How a Ballet Is Made.* London: Golden Gallery Press. A complete account of how a ballet is put together.

ROBERT, GRACE: *The Borzoi Book of Ballets.* Alfred A. Knopf, Inc. A description of ballets performed by American ballet companies.

SEYMOUR, MAURICE: *Ballet Portraits.* Pellegrini & Cudahy. Photographs of famous dancers.

SPARGER, CELIA: *Anatomy and Ballet.* The Macmillan Co. A technical book for dancers about the correct use of the body in ballet. Photographs, x-ray pictures and drawings illustrate the text.

STREATFEILD, NOEL: *Ballet Shoes.* Random House. A story about three girls in London who study the ballet.

WYNDHAM, LEE: *Slipper Under Glass.* Longmans, Green & Co. A story about a young ballet dancer.

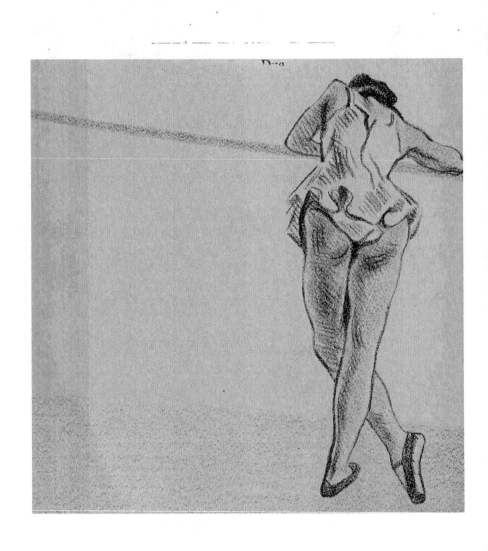

## DATE DUE

| | | |
|---|---|---|
| DE 1 75 | | |
| NO 25 76 | | |
| JY 17 78 | | |
| OCT 28 '81 | | |
| | | |
| | | |
| | | |
| | | |
| | | |
| | | |
| | | |
| | | |
| | | |
| | | |
| | | |
| | | |
| GAYLORD | | PRINTED IN U.S.A. |

CPSIA information can be obtained
at www.ICGtesting.com
Printed in the USA
LVHW021740120423
744164LV00004B/239